I0478473

ASTHMA THERAPY REGULATION

BY
AFIYA ANSARI

CONTENT

KEYWORDS: pediatrics, asthma, allergens, pollution, habitat, microclimate, diagnostic algorithm and treatment, treatment efficiency, advanced management.

INTRODUCTION

Asthma is a chronic disease of the air passages, common in all ages and considered as one of the most common chronic disease of children. The prevalence of asthma in children ranges between 10-15% and about 60% of asthmatic patients are diagnosed in childhood.

It is believed that asthma is a complex chronic inflammatory syndrome characterized by obstruction of airflow in the airway inflammation of chronic airway remodeling their walls, airway hyperreactivity to nonspecific stimuli and exacerbation episodes of airway obstruction causing respiratory symptoms specific mainly respiratory dyspnea and wheezing [1].

Understanding the pathogenesis of asthma has undergone major changes over the years, moving from the understanding of asthma as the primary condition airway caliber concept of immunity airway dysfunction that leads to chronic inflammation and structural abnormalities. The asthmatic children infiltration of mast cells was observed, eosinophils, CD4 + T cells (Th2), and Th17 airway walls, even in the case of mild or no symptoms severity [2]. Airway epithelium is the first line of interaction with the atmosphere, with the protective barrier. Recent studies suggest immunogenic and immunomodulatory functions of bronchial epithelium [2].

In asthma and recurrent respiratory symptoms are variable with significant impact on quality of life. The interaction between clinical, functional and biological symptoms causes clinical manifestations of asthma severity and response to treatment [3].

As a chronic inflammatory disease of the upper airways, asthma is influenced by the interaction of genetic and environmental factors, mediated by epigenetic field that studies the heritable changes in phenotype mitotic (changes in gene expression), without direct changes occurring DNA sequences. Creating new opportunities to advance original concepts on the mechanism of gene-environment interactions and to review the existing theories on asthma disease [4].

Asthma is common in children and adolescents, in part because of a higher incidence of allergies in these ages. The incidence of asthma has increased dramatically since 1970, the largest increase being in urban areas in developed countries, the trend followed in developing countries. According to WHO asthma occur at all ages but often begins in childhood. It is a disease characterized by recurrent attacks of breathlessness and wheezing, which vary in severity and frequency from person to person and even the same individual seizures may occur from hour to hour or day to day [5].

In spite of improved knowledge about the pathophysiology of asthma and the increased availability of new and safer drugs, mortality from this disease had an overall increase in the last 30 years [6].

Air pollution in the free atmosphere and in enclosed spaces remains an important public health problem, being responsible for exacerbation of preexisting respiratory or slowing growth and normal functioning of the lung in children as well as a potential cause in the development of asthma in this age [7]

Function of the dimensional spectrum of air pollutants (Fig.1) are affected different regions of the respiratory tract (Fig.2).

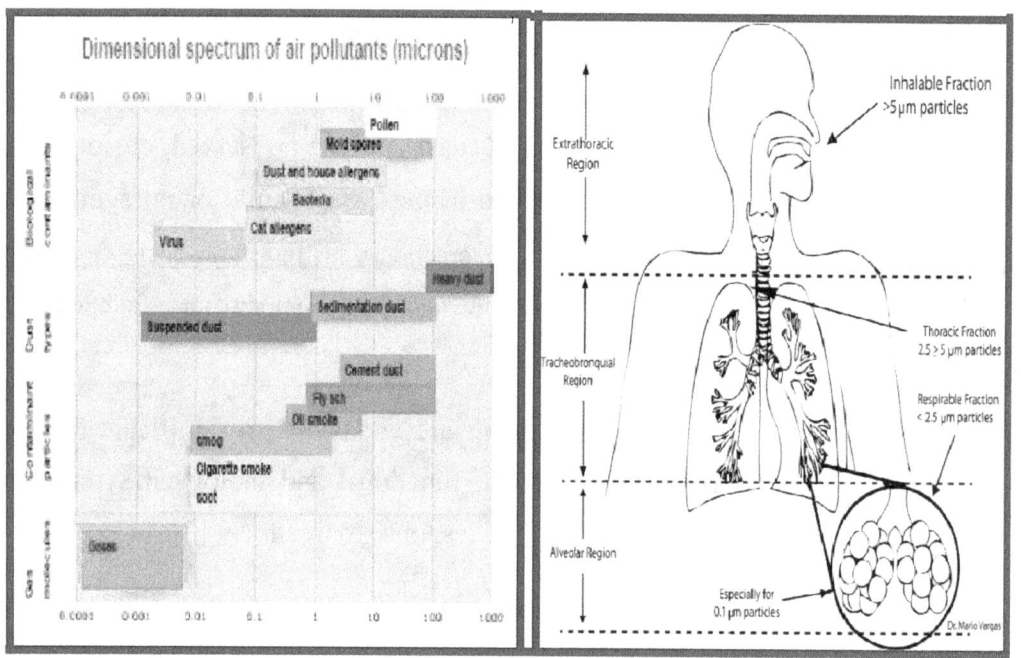

Fig.1. Dimensional spectrum of air pollutants **Fig.2.** Regional deposition of air particles [8]

The daily exposure to air pollution both in free atmosphere and indoor is associated with an increased risk of asthma in childhood. Even at low concentrations, the pollutants present in the air either in the form of particulate matter (PM) as well as in the form of gas (O_3 ozone, nitrogen dioxide NO_2, SO_2 sulfur dioxide, nitrogen oxides NO_x, carbon monoxide CO, volatile organic compounds VOC etc.) have a negative impact on respiratory health [8],[9]. In the urban areas may be responsible for adverse health effects and exacerbation of asthma pediatric which necessarily involves establishing effective measures to improve air quality by limiting pollutant sources in the free atmosphere and optimizing ventilation in enclosed spaces [10].

The microclimate, defined as all climatic conditions (temperature, humidity, wind) specific to small spaces is a result of interaction with the built environment area (housing, schools, etc.) is also a very important element in the analysis of asthmatic disease in children especially in terms of extreme weather events (heat waves, storms, etc.) [11], [12]. The climate at local and regional level can affect both the biological and chemical pollutants in the atmosphere and interior spaces [13], [14].

Under conditions of poor hygiene habitats robust regulatory mechanisms are needed to control individuals predisposed to developing allergies and asthmatic diseases. It has been shown that in such hygienic conditions and without access to clean running water for the first three years of life children have developed in the following years increased levels of spontaneous production of interleukin IL-10, which is attributed to high microbial exposure [15].

In recent years, there have been considerable advances in epidemiological studies, experimental and clinical asthma and respiratory allergies in children. Through recent investigations on epidemiological trends, risk factors and prevention of pediatric asthma and allergic diseases have been developed new concepts of immunology and pediatric allergy [16].

This doctoral thesis is divided into two main parts: general part, which includes current state of knowledge in the pediatric asthma field and personal study, which includes both research on the monitoring of particulate matter pollution in urban areas (Bucharest and Rosiori de Vede) as well as the assessment of asthma development in a group of children included in the study, treated with different classes of asthma drugs and its correlation with pollutant factors in the area and in the family environment.

CHAPTER 1. PRESENT STAGE OF CHILDREN ASTHMA KNOWLEDGE

This general part of the thesis treats in detail the most important scientific knowledge about asthma in children and presents a complex problem of disease from asthma definition , brief history , epidemiology , presenting epidemiological data in children, factors that trigger disease and chronic infection (genetic predisposition environmental factors) , asthma as chronic progressive disease (bronchial wall remodeling , chemical mediators involved in the pathogenesis of asthma, and asthma link between gut microbiota) , the differential diagnosis of asthma in children, asthma triggers (allergens , irritants respiratory diseases respiratory viral) , new guidelines for diagnosis and treatment of pediatric asthma , non- pharmacological management of asthma in children (control environment , spirometry , asthma diary and questionnaire assessment of asthma , asthma action plans). Have not been forgotten the methods for either chronic inflammation in asthma evaluation (determination of nitric oxide - NO in exhaled air, eosinophilic cationic protein). An important chapter is devoted to the pharmacological management of asthma in which the current data on the pharmacology of asthma control medication to the child (inhaled corticosteroids, beta2-adenomimetice with long-acting, leukotriene modifiers, antihistamines H1, xanthine derivatives - theophylline therapy, anti-IgE), prophylactic medication crisis (mast cell degranulation inhibitor - cromolyn and nedocromil).

Also is presented pharmacological and asthma rescue medication (beta2-adrenomimetice with short-acting, anticholinergic corticosteroids oral and parenteral). Are addressed issues related to the treatment of asthma induced by exercise, emergency treatment of acute asthma and immunotherapy in asthma in children (outpatient and hospital) and immunotherapy. In a synthetic way are described new therapeutic targets in asthma on the progress of research on the links and pathways involved in asthma pathogenesis and gene therapy basis. General part ends with outcome data of asthma in children and future perspectives

CHAPTER 2. PERSONAL STUDY

In this doctoral thesis, the study protocol for analysis of asthma incidence exacerbations in children asthma under the influence of environmental conditions (air pollution, microclimate and habitat, dwellings characteristics of investigated subjects) consisted of standardized questionnaires, medical examination and evaluation of these environmental conditions. Additional questionnaire focused on current symptoms and history of respiratory diseases investigated subjects and their families. The main investigated pollutans were Particle Materials PM2.5 şi PM10 during 2011-2012 period and also for previous years both in the metropolitan area of Bucharest as well as in Roşiori de Vede town, placed in the South-Eastern part of Romania. I have presented the evidence of the air pollutants effects on asthma patients among children, studies that have focused on the analysis of limitations of induced respiratory capacity and the efficiency of applied asthma treatment.

I analyzed the way in which the whole living conditions, dwelling, psychosocial influenced the evolution of asthmatic children treated for a period of one year. Of the habitat definitions I chose the biological definition: 1) all conditions of life offered by a biotope, ecotop; 2) The human ecosystem element consists of environmental factors and the psychosocial factors.

The objectives of asthma therapy in children include improved quality of life (normal physical activity). The specific objectives of treatment are to reduce inflammation, improve pulmonary function, reduce the clinical symptoms, reduce crises and therefore reduce hospitalizations, visits to emergency departments, absenteeism from school. Non-pharmacologic management strategies include avoidance of allergens, allergens and pollutants environmental assessment, patient education, allergy tests, regular monitoring of lung function and use of asthma management plan, asthma control tests, peak flow meters and diaries asthma. The achievement of the therapeutical objectives reduces direct and indirect costs of asthma [5].

2.1. STUDY MOTIVATION AND WORK HYPOTHESES

Asthma is considered the most common chronic disease of childhood with multifactor aspect where it is difficult to distinguish between causes and triggers. Infantile asthma prevalence has increased alarmingly in the last 30 years in Romania to children aged between 13 and 14 years, which are correlated with low air quality, exposure to allergens inside homes and stressful lifestyle [17]. Frequent pediatric asthma exacerbations are biggest stress for the patient, family and healthcare.

Although there is now a growing concern in the European authorities for the identification and study of risk factors and the chronic respiratory allergic diseases being underway at least two European programs for the prevention of asthma: Finnish and European program PAPA program (Prevention of Asthma, Prevention of Allergy), coordinated by the WHO Centre in Montpellier, with remarkable results, in Romania there is no consensus regarding the prevalence of pediatric asthma, but existing data show that the prevalence of asthma is higher in urban than in rural areas, morbidity being influenced by the lack of diagnosis and inadequate treatment.

The research aimed the detection of those correction factors which could bring the patient out of danger in the area of safety and contribute to improving pulmonary function in the long term. Due to the fact that long-term treatment of asthma is sometimes with the use of various types of medicines and the temporal variation of the intensity due to asthma in children is under the influence of many endogenous and exogenous factors, the adherence to the therapy is difficult to be handled in the management of asthma in children.

2.2. AIMS AND OBJECTIVES OF PERSONAL STUDY

In the personal study, I proposed to evaluate the influence of atmospheric pollution, climate and microclimate and habitat on patients response to treatment, to achieve and maintain asthma control, while identifying and correcting of those poor prognostic factors (exposure to a powerful allergy to pollutants inside the home as well - smoke, mold, dust mites, pet epithelia, presence of comorbidities of allergic respiratory and skin, as well as those non-allergic, obesity). I have decided to increase patient adherence to treatment and may improve result of the antiasthmatic treatment in children. There have also been monitored the side effects of chronic anti-inflammatory therapy.

The main objectives of this study are:

1. Establishing diagnostic strategy in asthma in children.

2. The evaluation of spirometric parameters (FEV 25% and MEF25%) and pulseoximetry in children from urban intensive pollution zones compared with patients from less polluted environment (rural).

3. Assessment of pediatric asthma exacerbations number function of pollution, microclimate and the habitat.

4. Evaluation IgE in studied patients, depending on the level of air pollution, microclimate and the habitat.

5.The correlation between C-reactive protein and stage of treatment with inhaled corticosteroids efficiency

6.The assessment of cigarette smoke influence (active or passive smoking) on the development of asthma and effectiveness of drug treatment.

7. The assessment of atmospheric pollution with particulate matter PM in urban areas Roşiori de Vede and Bucharest compared to rural areas.

8. Establishing of effective prevention and education measures of patients included in the study group

2.3. MATERIALS AND METHODS

This study was performed in the Department of Pediatrics of the Hospital Caritas from Rosiori de Vede, in Teleorman County , Romania, during February 2011 - February 2012, being a prospective study that was conducted in accordance with the Declaration of Helsinki entitled - Ethics and Epidemiology: International Guidelines, published by the Council for International Organizations of Medical Sciences. Recruitment of patients was made based on the study protocol approved by the Ethics Committee of UMF Craiova .

In the study entered a group of 55 patients aged 3 to 17 years of which 29 girls (52.72%) and 26 boys (47.27%), diagnosed with asthma prior to inclusion in the program are in treatment of asthma control, being compliance with the criteria for inclusion and exclusion set. Patients were monitored from the beginning of the study for 12 months with clinical and biological evaluation at 1 month, 3 months, 6 months and 12 months after enrollment and the whenever necessary. The study protocol was included in a computer algorithm that aimed the following anamnestico clinical, laboratory , parclinical and therapeutic aspects [20].

Were investigated epidemiological data, the number of exacerbations, respiratory functional parameters were monitored (FEV and MEF25%, pulse oximetry), monitored biological parameters (blood count, ESR, fibrinogen, blood eosinophilia and total serum IgE necessary to determine personal atopy); Allergy skin testing method prick skin test and specific IgE determination to aeroallergens and food allergens in allergic sensitization to establish support; complementary imaging investigations chest X-ray type or previous facial sinuses. Monitor the number of presentations to the family doctor or the emergency department and the number of hospital admissions in asthma exacerbation.

Antihistaminic treatment was applied according to the steps of severity and the intensity on a scale of 1-8, because presently severity of the asthma is classified on the basis of consensus intensity of treatment required for obtaining a good control of the disease [16], [21]. Inflammatory corticosteroid dose was further quantified in small, medium and large [22].

Monitoring the evolution was carried out at intervals of 1, 3, 6 and 12 months after study entry. Was developed a rigorous asthma management plan.

Have been clearly established investigation methods: history; clinical examination; paraclinical explorations (spirometry, pulseoximetry, total and specific IgE determination, determination of acute phase reactants erythrocyte sedimentation rate -ESR, fibrinogen and C-reactive protein); methods of statistical processing of data; methods for determining

PM air pollution (gravimetric used to measure particulate matter, urban test sites Rosiori de Vede and Bucharest).

In this doctoral thesis, the study protocol for the analysis in asthma exacerbations incidence in children under the influence of pollutant factors (air pollution, microclimate and habitat, housing characteristics of the investigated subjects) consisted of standardized questionnaires, medical examination and evaluation of these environmental conditions. Additional questionnaire focused on current symptoms of respiratory and personal historical data and family history correlated with asthma.

2.4. RESULTS

The performed researches during the study period established :

1) demographic and anthropometric characteristics of patients with asthma in the study group (55 children);

2) Past medical history, personal family history and habitat patients in the study group linked to pollution (combination asthma / dermatitis atypical-2 children combination asthma / allergic rhinitis, 9 children, combination asthma / allergic conjunctivitis, 4 children; combination asthma / rhinitis and allergic conjunctivitis, 2 children). 52 children with asthma have shown hypersensitivity to various pollutants in the atmosphere or IgE-mediated sensitization to multiple allergens. Meteorological conditions leading to the onset of asthma in the cold and fog (fog or moisture 5 children and 2 children cold) and 19 children with asthma (34.55%) showed hypersensitivity to particulate matter (dust) in the air. Inadequate habitat conditions met in children who had asthma smoke (4 children) by heating with wood or coal housing and a large number of children have shown hypersensitivity to the presence of mold or dampness in the home (17 representing 30.99%); A number of 14 children lived in a polluted environment with cigarette smoke (smoking one or both parents).

3) Secondary effects of inhaled corticosteroid therapy;

4) Therapies addressed differentially during the entire period of study patients;

5) The evolution of clinical, functional and biological parameters during the 12-month study (mean values evolution of body weight and height of children with asthma in the study group, body mass index, biological parameters, the mean values of spirometric indices and pulseoximetry, of the number of exacerbations of asthma

development by addressing the cabinet or ambulatory emergency services, the number of hospitalizations and severity of asthma);

6) The results of atmospheric pollution investigations regarding particle materials PM2.5 and PM10 concentrations in Bucharest metropolitan area [21], [22], [23], [24], [25], [26];

7) The results of asthma tests evaluation on subgroups of asthma children related to age, sex, residence, degree of environmental pollution (FEV evolution, MEF25%, pulseoximetry).

8) The results of the correlation between C-reactive protein and stage of treatment effectiveness of inhaled corticosteroids in asthma.

9) The results of the analysis between passive smoking of children with asthma and antiasthmatic stage of treatment effectiveness.

2.5. DISCUSSION OF RESULTS

The personal research study contents in two aspects, one related to the determination of particulate matter pollution in urban areas and one that evaluated evolution of of asthma in a group of children treated with different classes of asthma medication. Clinical experiences and dynamic tracking, through longitudinal studies of the development of asthma in children have shown that therapeutic interventions in the early stages of the disease are more effective. Also, a better knowledge and understanding of the pathogenic mechanisms responsible for the onset and progression of the disease are needed to optimize asthma care.

The paper highlighted that air pollution can exacerbate asthma in pediatric patients who have already condition and can also contribute to the initiation of new cases of asthma, that from biological point of view is plausible in the light of current theories of understanding of asthma as a complex disease with a variety of phenotypes.

This doctoral thesis focused on the objectives of asthma treatment in children for decreased mortality and improvement of life quality. The specific addressed objectives of the treatment are to reduce inflammation, improving lung function, reducing clinical symptoms, reduce crises and therefore reduce hospitalizations, visits to emergency departments, absences from school.

Non-pharmacologic management strategies include avoiding allergens, allergens and pollutants environmental assessment, patient education, allergy tests, regular monitoring of lung function and regularly use of asthma management plan, asthma control tests, peak flow meters and diaries asthma. Achieving therapeutic targets effectively contribute to reduce direct and indirect costs of pediatric asthma.

1) ***The analysis of demographic, anthropometric and biological characteristic features of the study group included:***

- The percentage distribution of the forms of asthma by severity in rural and urban environment (intermittent asthma, mild persistent asthma APU, medium persistent asthma APM, APS severe persistent asthma), (Fig.3);

- The distribution of patients by age (Fig.4);

- The distribution of study included patients by age and sex (Fig.5);

- The analysis of relation asthma obesity in the study group by plotting the values of body weight (kg) and height (cm) for the entire group of patients at baseline and end of study (Fig.6);

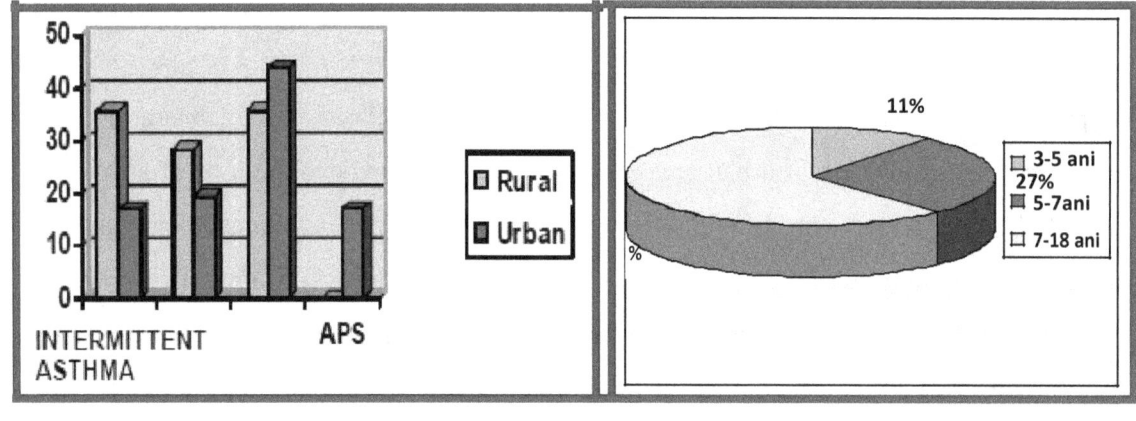

| Fig.3 | Fig.4 |

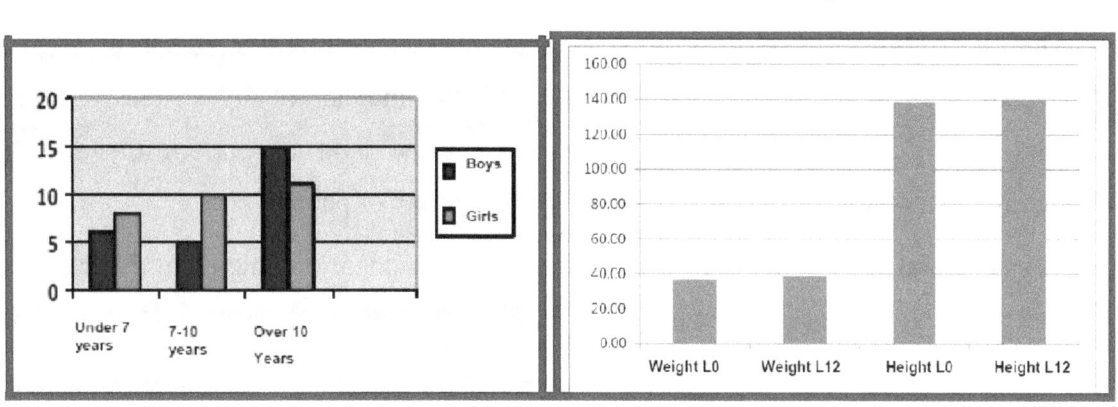

| Fig.5 | Fig.6 |

- The analysis of anthropometric parameters in patients treated with ICS and in patients not treated with ICS at baseline (L0) and end of the study (L12), (Fig.7);

- The analysis of the medical history of the study group (Fig.8);

- The analysis of the pathological heredocolaterale history of children with asthma in the lot;

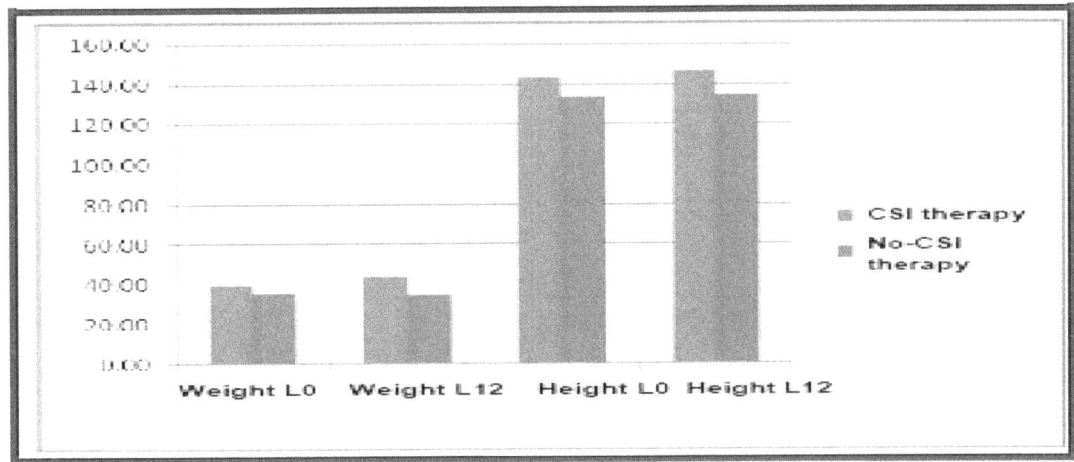

Fig.7

- Analysis of the personal pathological history of children with asthma in the lot, the distribution of patients according to the severity of asthma at enrollment (Figure 9); graphical representation of the severity of asthma (cases) by age and sex at study start (Fig. 10);

- positive family history analysis that has found more severe forms of asthma in children with predisposing genetic factors (family with parents, siblings with asthma or other allergic manifestations;

- Evolution of the of severity of asthma between the beginning and end of the study, to the whole group of patients (Figure 11); Distribution of patients after treatment carried out during the study (Fig.12);

- Treatment evolution for asthma patients included in the study (Fig.13).

- The analysis of spirometric parameters (Fig.14, Fig.15, Fig.16);

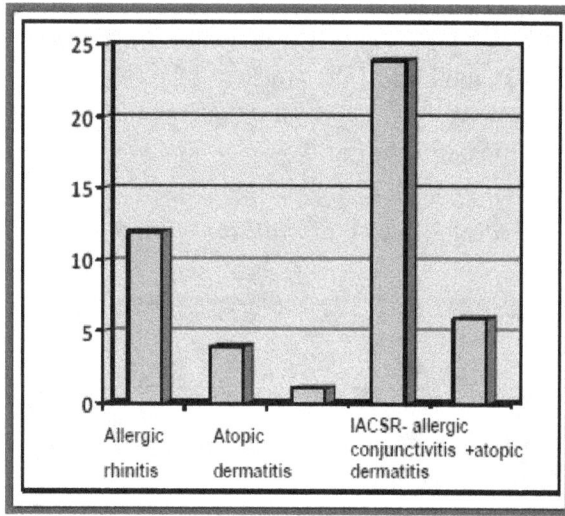

Fig.8

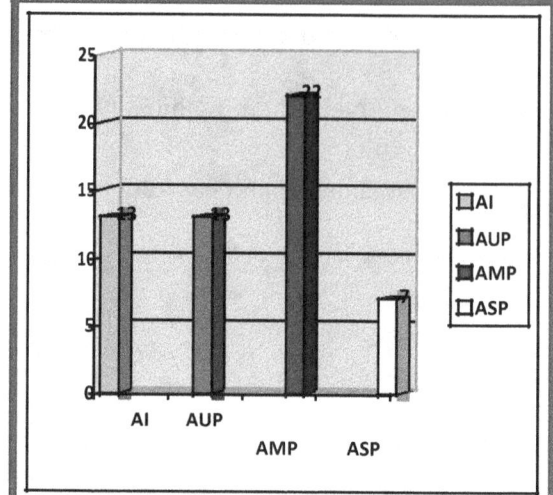

Fig.9

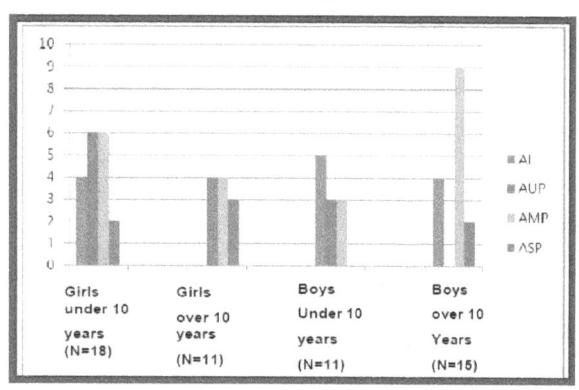

Fig.10

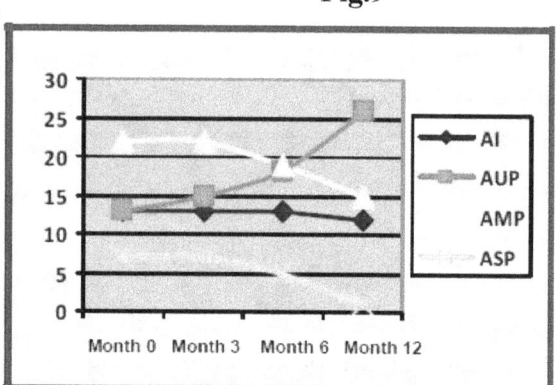

Fig.11

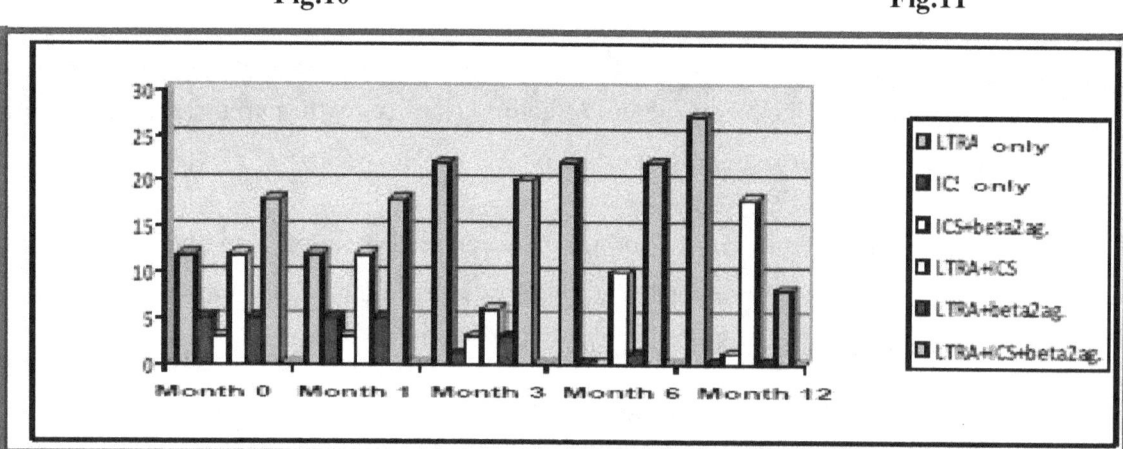

Fig.12

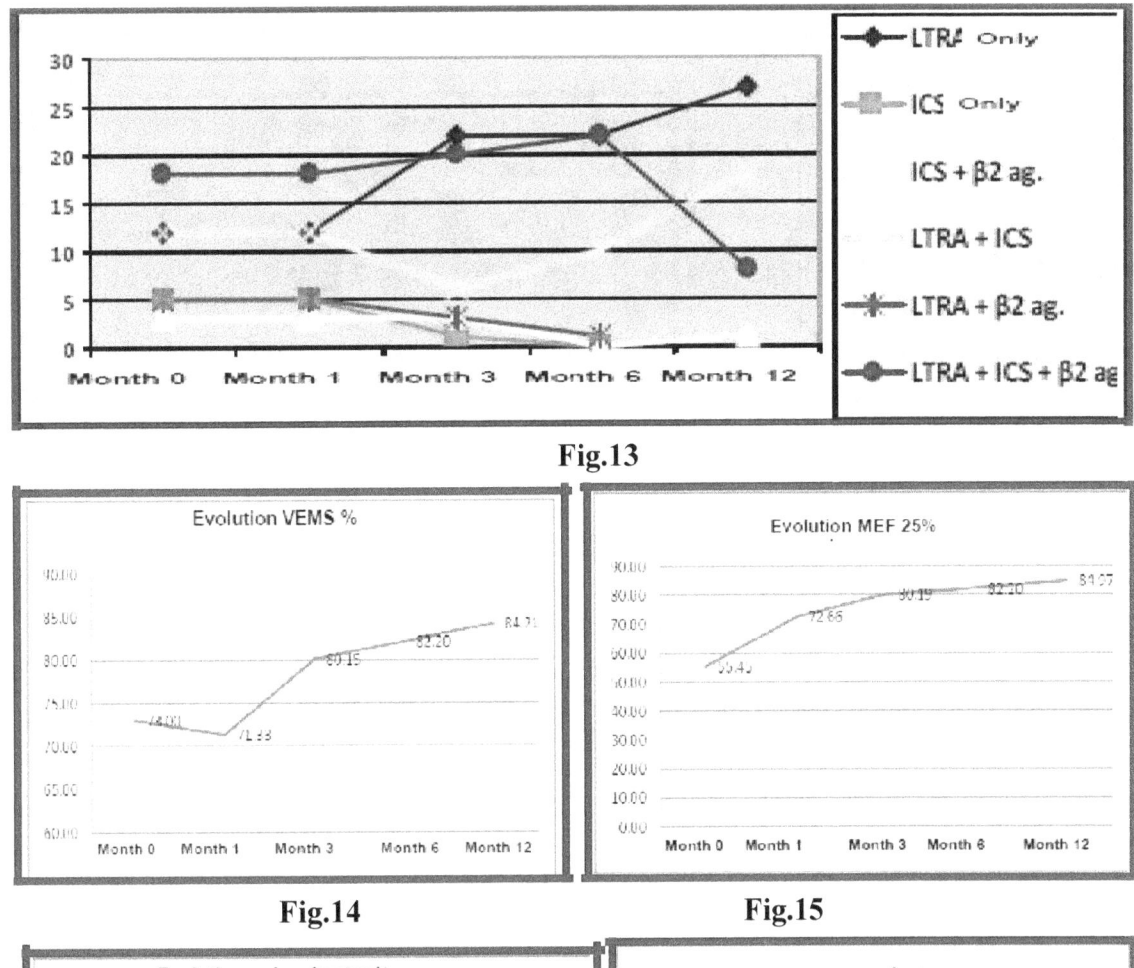

Fig.13

Fig.14

Fig.15

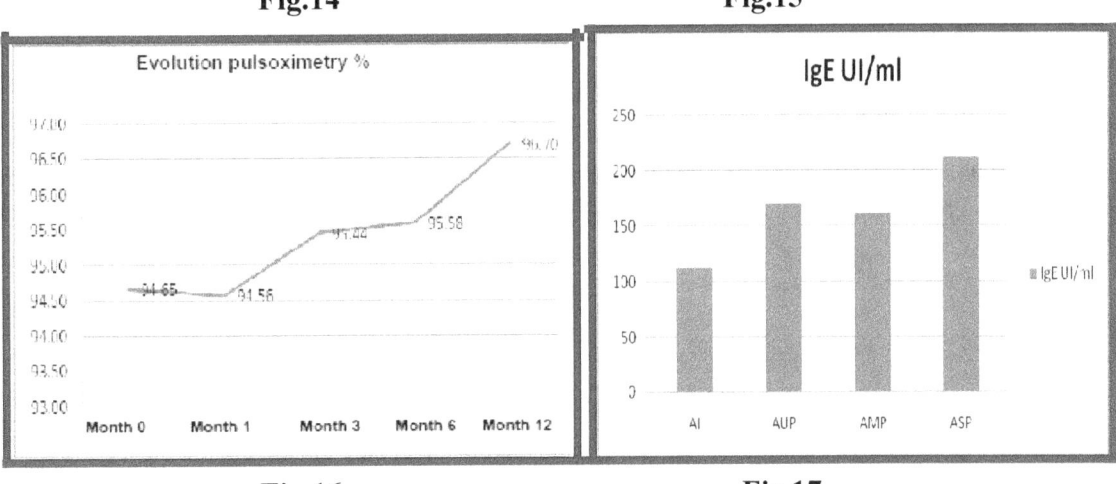

Fig.16

Fig.17

- The analysis of the IgE values evolution in the study group: at the beginning of the study (graphical representation of average IgE values depending on the severity of asthma -Fig.17; IgE values (average) by area of residence at study start, Fig.18), the graphical representation of the mean values of IgE to the whole group of patients (Fig.19); Evolution IgE values measured in the study group at baseline (month 0) and at the end of study ,month 12 (Fig.20).

- The analysis of ESR (Fig.21) and Fibrinogen parameters (Fig.22);

- Evolution of the number of exacerbations and the number of hospital admissions during the study (Fig.23 and Fig.24);

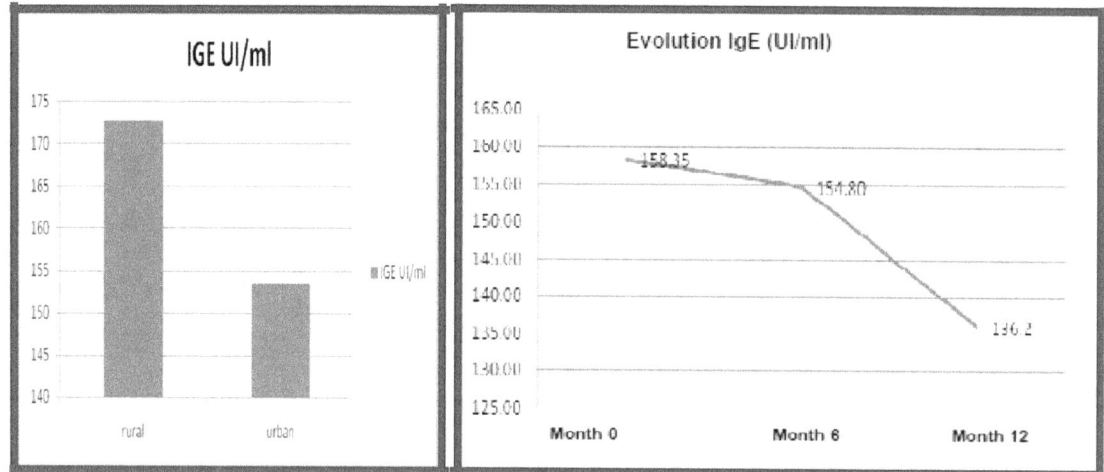

Fig.18   Fig.19

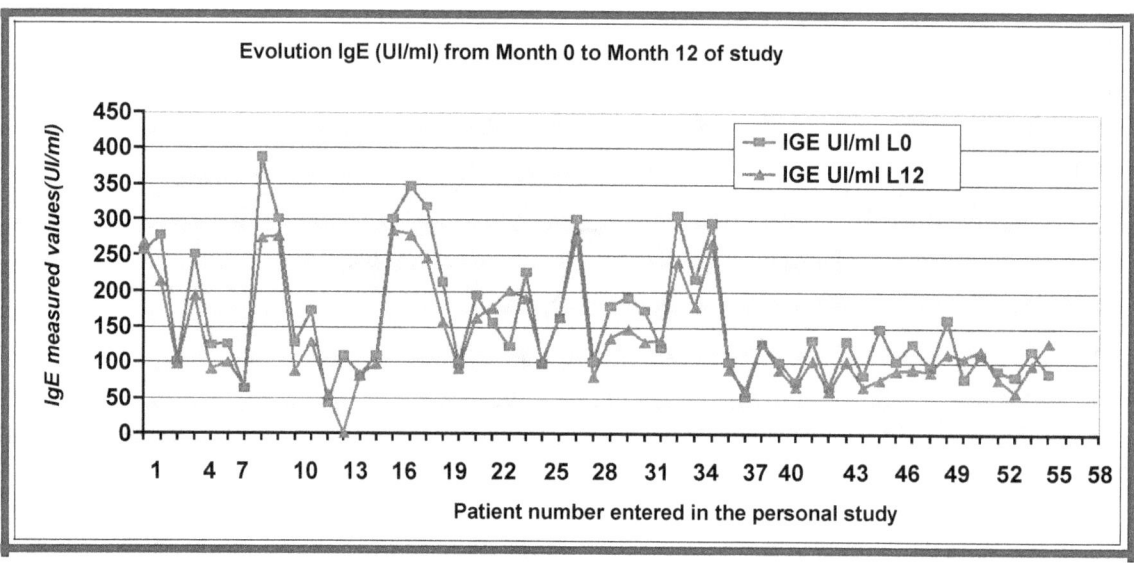

Fig.20

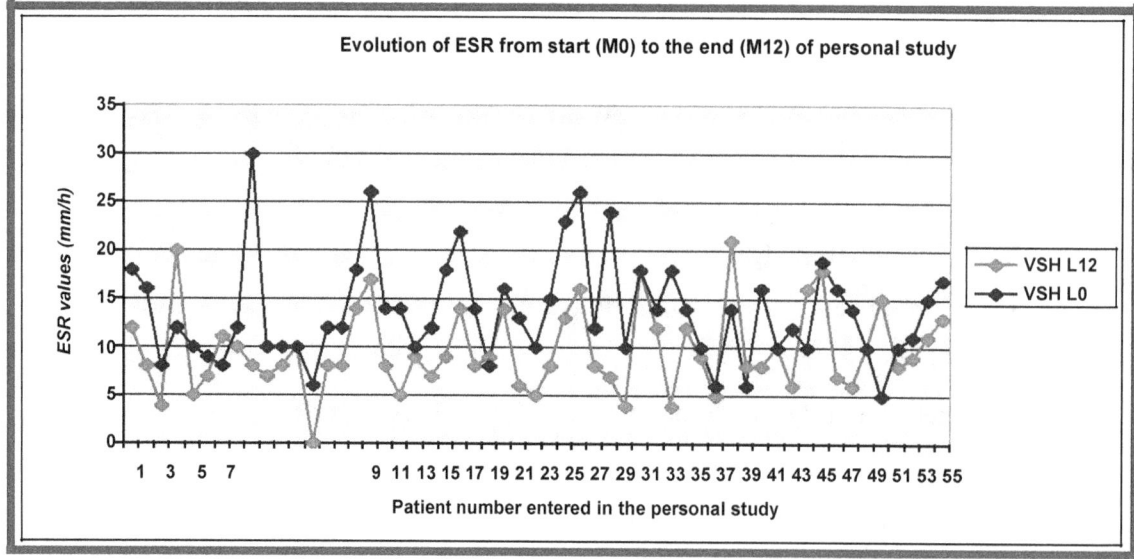

Fig.21

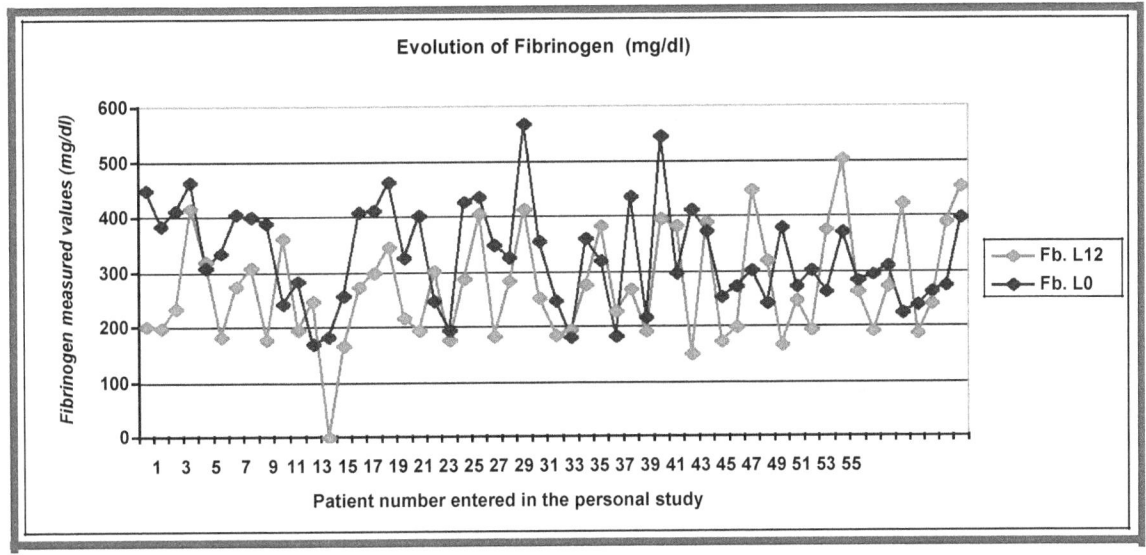

Fig.22

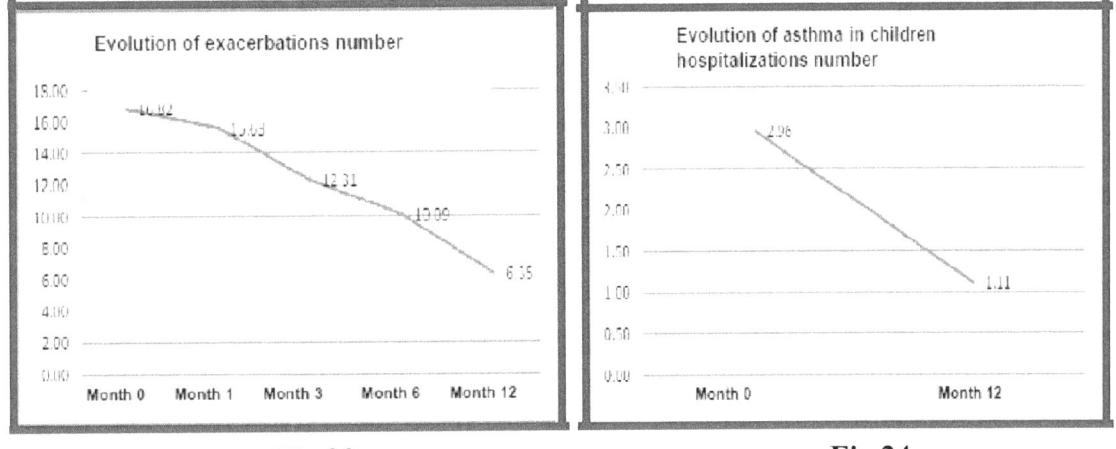

Fig.23   **Fig.24**

Administration of advanced treatments specific notably through the introduction inhaled corticosteroids and long-acting β-agonists for group of asthmatic children patients during the study helped the relieve of asthma clinical symptoms and reduce the frequency of severe exacerbations and improving actual test results that targeted evolution of favorable improvement in airway inflammation and infection and registered by a decrease in ESR -erythrocyte sedimentation rates in the month 12 monitored in comparison with month zero at the entry in the study.

It can be said that the anti-inflammatory action of prescribed medication for asthmatic children and adolescents throughout the study may counteract the negative respiratory effects of particulate matter PM pollution and toxic gases from urban environment, rural seasonal allergies and inside the homes pollution with cigarette smoke, carbon dioxide and micro-organisms.

2) **The analysis of asthma evolution through physiological parameters VEMS 25% , MEF 25% and SaO2 on subgroups of patients according to age, sex, residence place**

- Evolution of physiological parameters measured in subgroups of patients according to age (3-7 years and 8-17 years) between males and females, and between the urban and the rural showed that there are no significant differences between the two subgroups statistically track parameters (FEV, MEF25%, pulse oximetry) at times of assessment (at the beginning of the study, 1 month, 3 months, 6 months, 1 year). *So age and sex of the children were not factors influencing treatment response and that favorable development of spirometric parameters and pulseoximetry.*

- Evolution of physiological parameters measured in subgroups of patients according to area of residence (urban and rural) revealed significant differences statistically for all assessment times (baseline, 1 month, 3 months, 6 months, 1 year) between two subgroups, for FEV 25% (Fig. 25) in good agreement with literature [27], [28]. *The differences were attributed to the influence of air pollution. For MEF25% we obtained significant differences only for evaluations in the first months (0 and 1). (Fig.26). The analysis of pulseoximetry values obtained did not show statistically significant differences. Overall, the physiological parameter values were higher in patients from rural areas compared to urban ones, which demonstrates the negative influence of air pollution higher in the urban zones.*

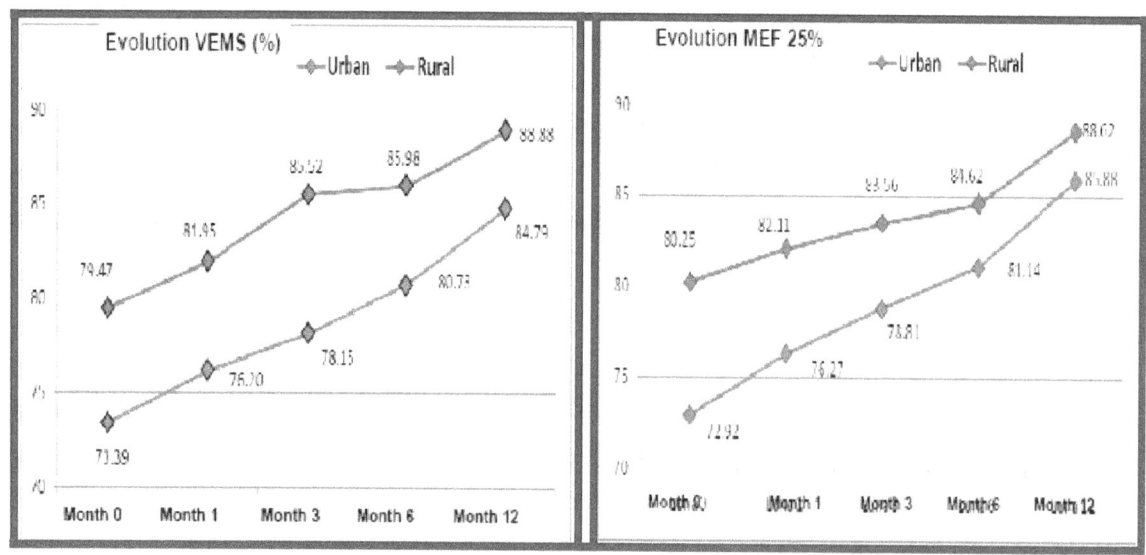

Fig.25   Fig.26

- The analysis of physiological parameters in subgroups of patients according to the factors of pollution classified into 3 major categories of pollution (without pollutants, smoking and industrial pollution parents) did not show significant differences. For FEV 25% and MEF 25% improvement of the differentiated between the three groups meets every 3 months monitoring, especially for MEF 25% when the group without pollution the average value is 83.59% compared to 78.32% in lot of pollution and 80.96% in the group with smoking parents. *Polluted environment conditions are also reflected in the analysis of the relationship between patient age and the age of the patient's asthma* (Fig. 27).

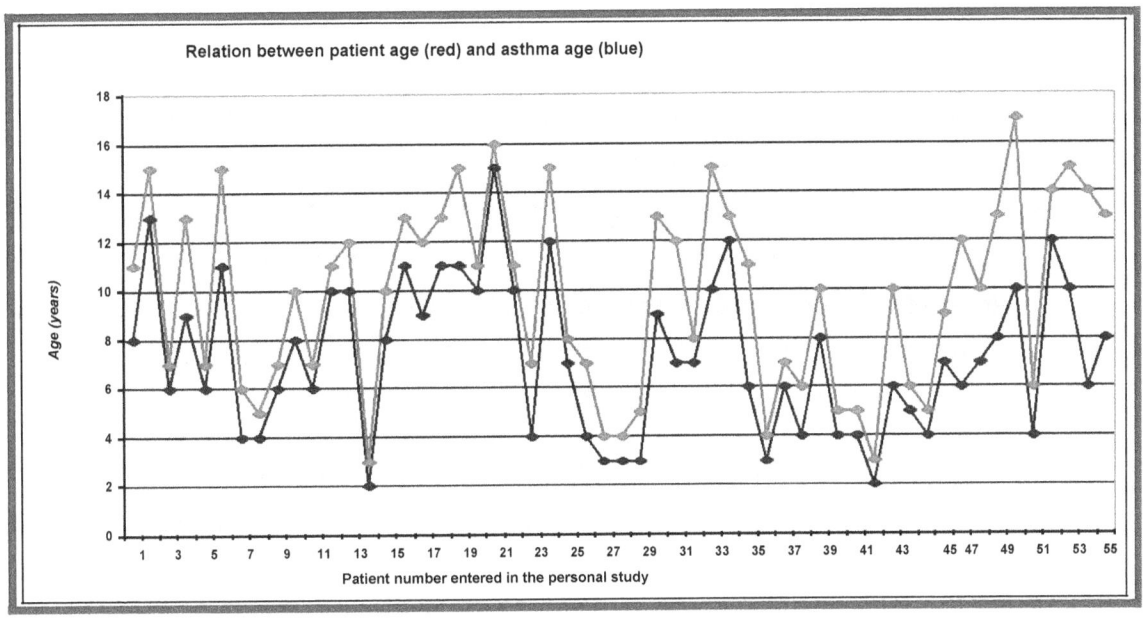

Fig.27

3) *The analysis of asthma evolution by Body Mass Index (BMI) at entry and exit of the study*

- According to epidemiological studies in the most recent literature, childhood obesity is closely correlated with asthmatic syndrome sometimes precedes asthma pediatric obesity [31], [32], [33]. From the investigations done in this study was confirmed that all patients in the study group analyzed body mass index falling into group "obesity" (1, 4, 6, 25, 29, 36, 41 and 51) live in the environment areas affected by pollution, but also characterized by inactivity and lack of exercise (Fig.28).

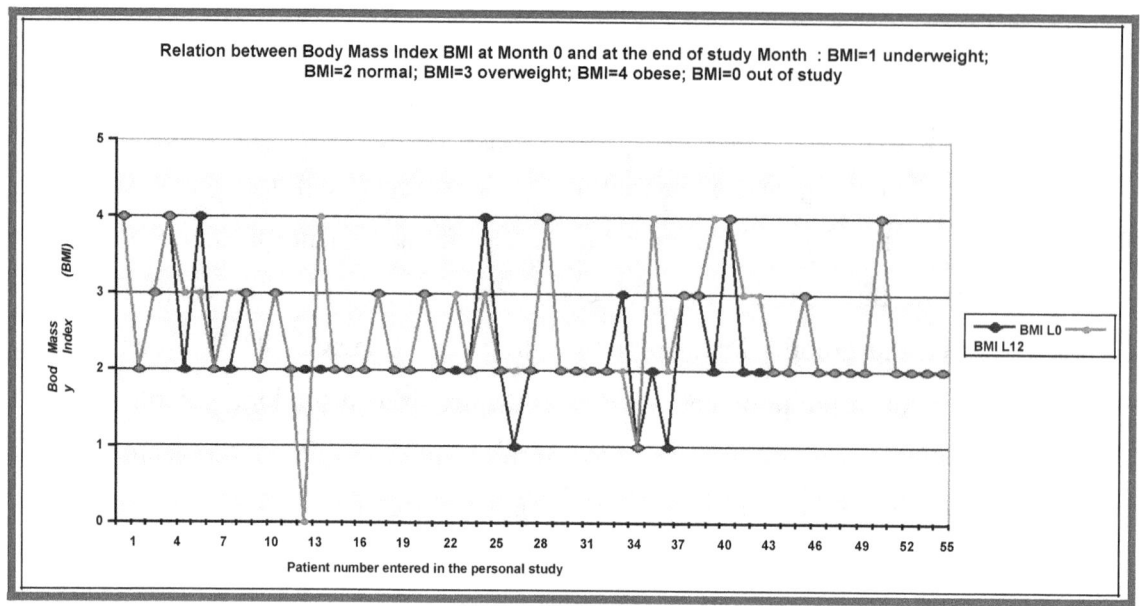

Fig.28

2.6. CONCLUSIONS ON THE STUDY RESULTS

1. The longitudinal clinical study on the relationship between air pollutants from both the outdoor environment as well as from indoor spaces (homes, schools) and asthma was conducted on a group of 55 children with asthma selected through rigorous inclusion and exclusion criteria in the pediatric Hospital Caritas in the town Rosiori de Vede and to obtain the written consent of parents or children to subordinate the treatment and monitoring criteria according to established protocol.

2. The study protocol for the analysis in asthma exacerbations incidence in children under the influence of air pollutants, climatic factors and habitat consisted of standardized questionnaires, clinical examination and paraclinical, pollution assessment and implementation of appropriate therapy for asthma control.

3. Children with asthma have been classified according to the severity of asthma according to the criteria the respiratory function and therapeutic criteria in accordance with existing international guidelines (intermittent asthma, mild persistent asthma, persistent asthma medium and severe persistent asthma).

4. Each child and parents have been trained on asthma monitoring, removal pollutant factors and the adherence to treatment.

5. The monitoring of asthma was performed at study entry, at 1, 3, 6 and 12 months and whenever was needed.

6. The assessment of of asthma evolution in relation to pollutants and complexity of treatment was conducted through spirometric measurements, pulseoximetry, allergy tests (total and specific IgE, skin prick tests as needed), biological samples (CRP, ESR, fibrinogen).

7. The values of total serum IgE at the beginning of the study were above the normal range in 60% of children in the group. Analyzing the total IgE for severe persistent asthma compared to those for other forms of asthma can be argued that the values of total IgE may be a predictive factor for severe persistent of asthma installation.

8. Through significant reduction of serum total IgE after 12 months of treatment and monitoring be claimed that they may also be a predictor of effectiveness of the treatment when it initially are increased.

9. The main investigated pollutants have been material particles PM2.5 and PM10 present both in the metropolitan area of Bucharest and the city Rosiori de Vede during 2011-2012, as well as for previous years .

10. High concentrations of pollutant aerosols present in urban and suburban areas of the city Roşiori de Vede, in some periods of the year, and in Bucharest (for children commuter schools in Bucharest) are responsible for direct and indirect effects on high risk asthmatic condition of the lot children.

11. Analyzed group presented a familial predisposition toward an unfavourable evolution of asthma due to poor outcome in terms of harmful environmental factors (pollution with PM, gas, inhaled allergens, etc.).

12. From analyzing of both personal history and family history background analysis have emerged a number of risk factors some of which can be removed in order to avoid repeated exacerbations.

13. Of those 55 children with asthma 25.45% have had passive smoking as a risk factor in the habitat, and their age was less than 7 years.

14. The study shows that the change of risk factors as family environment with smokers, improving living conditions and hygiene (removal of mold, mildew) has a significant positive impact on the evolution of of asthma.

15. It was noted the presence of some more severe forms of asthma in patients with a hereditary predisposition and atopy.

16. C-reactive protein is a biomarker for assessing asthma control in children. It was noted

a correlation between the presence of PCR in blood and the development of asthma therapy.

17. Obesity as a factor of personal pathology of asthma negatively influenced the evolution of children asthma, with the need to use some higher treatment steps.

18. Although comparative values were not statistically significant, however, FEVS and MEF25% and pulseoximetry positive evolved in the group with environmental pollution moved in the 12 months to lower values compared to the group without pollution.

19. The most important environmental factors for asthmatics children in the study group are air pollutants from open or indoor spaces where children live , exposure to air allergens, parental smoking and socioeconomic conditions.

20. The changes of the climatic conditions (high temperatures, high concentrations of CO_2, intense periods of rainfall, humidity changes) determined the increased frequency of asthma exacerbations.

21. The permanent monitoring, education of parents and children to avoid exacerbations and as far as possible removal of asthma triggers led to an improvement in children from the lot quality of life, reduce absenteeism from school and the good psycho-somatic development .

CHAPTER 3. GENERAL CONCLUSIONS, ORIGINALITY ELEMENTS AND FUTURE PERSONAL RESEARCH PERSPECTIVES
GENERAL CONCLUSIONS

1. Asthma, the most common chronic disease of childhood is a heterogeneous disease in which grades of severity and their evolution are variable depending on the patient. It is very difficult the step to patients severity classification. From the analysis of the lot of 55 children with asthma results important differences in asthma severity interpretation whether the assessment is conducted strictly according to symptoms and alteration of respiratory function parameters, or if the account is considered the intensity of treatment required to control symptoms.

2. The study makes a major contribution to the establishment of phenotypic features in the forms of severe asthma in children with atopy family of the disadvantaged social environments, multisensitivities (dust, mold and animal epithelia), which frequently associate rhinitis, allergic rhinosinusitis and allergic conjunctivitis as comorbidity, flammable phenotype characterized by the presence of polymorphonuclear respiratory

secretions and an obstructive functional pattern fixed distally to the breath.

3. In the personal study could be identified the unfavorable evolution of asthma risk factors, evaluated for each step of severity and graded according to the level of influence: impact factors (viral respiratory infections or microbial adherence to treatment) factors with a medium impact (allergic rhinitis, obesity, cigarette smoke exposure and atopy family environmental conditions) and low impact factors (sex, multisensitivity and age). The most important environmental factors in the study group are air pollutants, allergen exposure, parental smoking and socioeconomic conditions.

4. Factors related to the occurrence of asthma in childhood include atopy, sex, genotype, prenatal factors, higher age at first episode of wheezing, asthma in one or both parents and allergic rhinitis but also environmental factors like as allergen exposure, smoking active and passive irritants and pollutants, diet and obesity and socioeconomic factors.

5. Regular monitoring of the growth process should be a fundamental assessment of physical development in children with asthma. This monitoring should not be limited to measuring height and body weight, but should include an extensive range of somatic measurements to increase the accuracy of evaluation, ex. body mass index. This approach increases the probability that physical development disorders are detected early so that it can be initiated rehabilitation and the effectiveness of treatment can be assessed.

6. The constant application of protocols for diagnosis and treatment according to the clinical form of asthma in children external and the intervention on external pollutant factors through the education of parents and children led to very valuable results, viewed in marked remission of asthma in 33 patients after 6 months of treatment.

7. The study results show that total IgE approached and CRP- C Reactive Protein significantly correlated with the severity of asthma, and such information may allow prediction of the severity of illness in children with extremely high serum total IgE in order to change the disease course by such an intelligent therapeutic approach in order to reduce the number of hospitalizations and prevent disease persistence into adulthood.

8. In the study group we defined a subset of the phenotype "obese asthmatic child" and noticed the correlation between the two co-morbidities, the presence of systemic inflammation with local inflammation in the lung, and the negative development of asthma compared to non-obese asthmatics.

9. All patients in our study responded favorably to therapy with inhaled corticosteroids that which reconfirms the therapeutic efficacy of the ICS. Knowledge by the pediatrician of the progress in delimiting the fundamentals of pharmacology of glucocorticoids, especially transactivation and transrepression concepts and cofactor recruitment led to a better understanding of the molecular mechanisms by which glucocorticoids suppress inflammation and of necessity of this therapy. It is imperative to establish a school for parents to handle background therapy.

10. Although the findings of this study suggest that there is little difference between the effectiveness of a leukotriene receptor antagonist (LTRA) and an inhaled corticosteroid (ICS) as first-line therapy control between an LTRA and beta2-agonist long-action as add-on medication for ICS, caution is needed in interpreting these results.

11. Based on periodic medical examinations and the treatment with prescribed medications inhaled corticosteroid, antileukotriene, adrenomimetics type or combinations we analyzed the efficiency of applied treatment during one year of study, with assessments of the health of asthmatic children at intervals of 1 month, 3 months, 6 months and 12 months. The results of this study clearly show the efficiency of prescribed medication by the significant improvement of respiratory function in 53 (96,54%) asthmatic children entered the study (only 1 patient was poorly improved, and the other came out of the study).

12. Anti-asthmatic treatment associated administered with that of allergic comorbidities significantly improved respiratory functional parameters and quality of life by decreasing respiratory exacerbations and asthmatic crisis and hospitalizations in the study group.

13. This study highlighted the efficiency of asthma medication to children and teenagers during 1 year to decrease airway bronchial inflammations and specific respiratory infections in pediatric asthma syndrome manifested by improving ESR, fibrinogen and C-reactive protein values in the month 12 of monitoring compared with the zero month entry into the study.

14. It was highlighted the importance of atopy and genetic factors in influencing the level of severity of asthma in association with environmental factors, as risk factors for unfavorable evolution in asthma.

15. Early diagnosis and early therapeutic interventions are an essential element in achieving asthma control and perhaps even preventing it. Adherence to treatment of the

child and implicitly of the parents is another essential element in achieving asthma control therapy in children. Pediatric services must ensure effective training ways to parents.

16. Although it was observed that there are clear differences in severity of disease forms of asthma in children, have not yet been able precise prognostic shape phenotypes. But it is definite the influence of certain environmental factors which through their corrections due to control measures and environmental education can improve the asthma evolution.

17. Recently rapid advances were made in the treatment of asthmaas well as the appearance constantly of new medicines. It is important to improve symptoms while minimizing side effects of these drugs, which include disturbances of physical development. The presence of side effects is influenced by the the step of severity, the age of patients, and dosage. For the design of effective treatment protocols are essential additional studies on significant groups of asthmatic children.

18. Pediatric asthma therapeutic actions should aim not only to create wellbeing in asthma but also the use of new tools to predict risks and adopt the steps not only for the prevention of asthma exacerbations, but also for the prevention of early disease manifestations and through this to prevent evolution to severe asthma.

19. Through its results this doctoral thesis brings new contributions for the benefit of pediatric asthma management system in Romania, proposing development of a proper algorithm for diagnostic and therapeutic approach to family medicine and pediatric specialists.

20. Information and obtained results in this doctoral thesis are useful in identifying the risk of early asthma in children , applying the early intervention with the available therapies and conducting future studies in order to identify effective strategies to improve the asthma in children.

21. The physician should look at child asthma complexity together with all the factors that can influence severity, evolution and effectiveness of the treatment, so that the result shall be optimal regardless of its phenotype to know which environmental factors must be positively influenced .

22. Reducing the risk and perhaps even primary prevention of asthma remains an illusion, but it is the golden key of the herd management of asthma.

23. This doctoral thesis proposes the implementation of educational programs for parents of children with asthma who need to have sufficient knowledge to effectively manage asthmatic syndrome as well as for educators in schools and for asthmatic child himself.

24. Although we remarked a correlation between air pollution and exacerbation of asthma in children with asthma in city Roşiori de Vede can not be claimed clearly that heavy traffic or local sources of pollution are the main factors of poor evolution of asthma.

25. Free atmosphere and indoor air pollutants which are present in the early years of children are triggers of asthma symptoms leading to weak performance and a weaker response to anti-inflammatory therapy with inhaled corticosteroids and the inadequate development of the lungs .

26. Although in present research are highlighted sufficient evidence that air pollution (indoor or outdoor) favor the onset of asthma symptoms still presently can not be claimed definitely that air pollution is the main cause or direct in the increasing prevalence of asthma because asthma as a complex syndrome is influenced by many other factors as predisposing factors: age, sex, obesity, genetic factors; Respiratory infection with rhinovirus, influenza virus, respiratory syncytial virus, human metapneumovirus; behavioral factors (tobacco smoking); factors related to diet (some foods or medications).

27. From the analysis of the complex data obtained through this research regarding the influence of environmental factors on the effectiveness and antiasthmatic treatment of the disease can be suppositionated an interrelation between genetic, epigenetic and air pollution in asthma.

28. It is imperative to develop innovative management plans of pediatric asthma to manage asthma over time and facilitate decisions on interventions in order to maintain control leading to remission and prevention of disease exacerbations in children.

29. Is absolutely necessary to be taken effective and urgent measures by environmental management decision makers to reduce air pollutants with major implications for the prevalence of asthma in children and its incidence.

ORIGINALITY ELEMENTS OF DOCTORAL THESIS

- This is an original study, prospective and observational depth of a significant group of pediatric patients with different stages of asthma severity and different evolution stages, which facilitated outlining some sensible evolutionary trends under the influence of risk factors. The study covers the territory of a county area of Teleorman and can be very valuable because it establishes a local prevalence of asthma in children of about 7% -9%, data that coincide with data reporting nationwide.

- The modern Interpretation of pediatric asthma severity according to the level required to achieve therapeutic touch control opened a new perspective targeting impact related morbidity of this disease. The study is of considerable value to practitioners of family medicine and pediatric specialists by quantifying local environmental factors responsible for the disease.

- The monitoring of asthmatic patients through comprehensive tests of quality of life related to environmental risk factors, climatic and habitat, use of modern techniques including modern spirometric techniques for assessment of obstruction of the small airways and better classification of patients in the severity steps facilitates optimal differently treatment .

- Through the strategy of pediatric asthma control, prediction and prevention as well as in clinical practice conducted therapies addressed, this doctoral thesis contributes to the development of research on pediatric asthma in the Romania.

- It is proposed an algorithm for the approach by practitioners of new cases of asthma on minimal diagnostic investigations.

FUTURE PERSONAL RESEARCH PERSPECTIVES

- The implementation of allergy investigation in the pregnant women in order to reduce the development of allergic diseases in children with genetic predispositions therefore identifying the family history of allergies;

- Application of special measures for dispensary atopic risk children within primary prevention programs in family doctor's office in collaboration with the pediatrician and allergist to avoid exposure to risk factors;

- Identify characteristics of different forms of phenotypic biomarkers characteristic to asthma different clinical evolutive forms and implementing frequent monitoring airway inflammation, by measuring exhaled NO. Will be identified the different phenotypes of pediatric asthma starting with the non-allergic infant.

- Permanent monitoring of children with asthma and counting therapeutic interventions in the asthma control through the introduction of personal health booklets;

- The implementation on the possible new techniques for the determination of virological and bacteriological for relational interpretations viral infections - host-asthma;

- Improving the patient access to allergy clinics and their integration into specialized educational programs of medical personnel responsible of management of asthma in children. It is imperative to organize the educational schools for parents.

Through control strategy and approach to clinical practice and specific therapies in the pediatric asthma investigations within this study, prediction and prevention of asthma prevalence in children, the thesis contributes substantially to the development of scientific research on pediatric asthma in the Romania in relation with air pollution conditions and climate changes.

Selective References

[1]Plesca Doina, Hurduc Victoria, Ioan Iulia, Bădărău Anca. Chronic cough in childhood: a clinical and therapeutic approach, Part II, Therapeutics, Pharmacology and clinical Toxicology, (2009), 13(3) 287-294.

[2]Bartemes K.R., Kita H. Dynamic role of epithelium-derived cytokines in asthma, Clinical Immunology, (2012), 143, 222–235.

[3]Chang Ch. Asthma in Children and Adolescents: A Comprehensive Approach to Diagnosis and Management. Clinic Rev Allerg Immunol. (2012), 43:98–137.

[4]World Health Organization Fact Sheet Fact sheet No 307: "Asthma", (2011). [5]Lewis TC, Robins ThG, Mentz B Graciela et al. Air pollution and respiratory
symptoms among children with asthma: Vulnerability by corticosteroid use and reSidence area. Science of the Total Environment, (2013), 448: 48–55.

[6]Holgate ST. A Brief History of Asthma and Its Mechanisms to Modern Concepts of Disease Pathogenesis. Allergy Asthma Immunol Res., (2010), July; 2(3): 165–171.

[7]Möller W, Felten K, Sommerer K et al. Deposition, retention, and translocation of ultrafine particles from the central airways and lung periphery. Am. J. Respir. Crit. Care Med., (2008), 177: 426–32.

[8]Macintyre EA, Brauer M, et a.,GSTP1 and TNF Gene Variants and Associations between Air Pollution and Incident Childhood Asthma: The Traffic, Asthma and Genetics (TAG) Study., (2014), Jan .

[9]Kelly FJ, Fussell JC, Air pollution and airway disease, clinical & Experimental Allergy, (2011) 41, 1059–1071.

[10]Rosenlund M, Forastiere F, Porta D, De Sario M, Badaloni C, Perucci CA., Traffic-related air pollution in relation to respiratory symptoms, allergic senSitization and lung function in schoolchildren.Thorax,(2009), 64:573–80.

[11]O,,ConnorTG, Neas L, Vaughn B, et al. Acute respiratory health effects of air pollution on children with asthma in US inner cities. J Allergy Clin Immunol, (2008),121:1133-9.

[12]Sheehan WJ, Rangsithienchai PA, Wood RA et al. Pest and allergen exposure and abatement in inner-city asthma: a work group report of the American Academy of Allergy, Asthma & Immunology Indoor Allergy/Air Pollution Committee. J Allergy Clin Immunol

,(2010),125:575–581.

[13]Bernstein, J.A., Alexis, N., Bacchus, H., Bernstein, I.L., Fritz, P., Horner, E., Li, N., Mason, S., Nel, A., Oullette, J., Reijula, K., Reponen, T., Seltzer, J., Smith, A. and Tarlo, S.M. (2008), The health effects of non-industrial indoor air pollution, J. Allergy Clin. Immunol. 121, 585–591.

[14]Hulin M., Caillaud D., AnneSi-Maesano I., (2010), Indoor air pollution and childhood asthma: variations between urban and rural areas, Indoor Air 20, 502–514.

[15]GINA_Report _March (2013). Global strategy for asthma management and prevention. NIH

publication no. 02-3659 (updated 2012). 2012. National Institutes of Health/National Heart, Lung, and Blood Institute. Available on the GINA webSite www.ginasthma.org.

[16]Simpson CR, Sheikh A. Trends in the epidemiology of asthma in England: a national study of 333,294 patients.J R Soc Med.,(2010) ,103(3):98-106.

[17]European Environment and Health Information System. Prevalence of asthma and allergies in childen. Fact Seet NO 3.1.May (2007), CODE RPG3-AIR-E1.

[18] **Didă Mariana Rodica,** Studiul privind eficiența tratamentului astmului la copii in relatie cu poluanții atmosferici din zone urbane Si rurale, "Al Xi lea Congres National de Pediatrie, cu participare internationala, (2013), 25-28 sept,Targu Mures , Romania,e-poster.

[19] GINA Reports (2010), Global Strategy for Asthma Management and Prevention, http://www. ginasthma. org.

[20]Krishnan J., Bender B., Wamboldt F., Szefler S., Adkinson N. F., Zeiger R., Wise R., Bilderback A., Rand C. Adherence to inhaled corticosteroids: An ancillary study of the Childhood Asthma Management Program clinical trial, J Allergy Clin Immunol, (2012), 129,112-8.

[21]**Didă Mariana Rodica**, Maria Zoran, Long-term exposure to outdoor urban air pollution with particulate matter for prevalence of asthma symptoms, Proceeding BalkanPhySical Union 8 Conference, (2012), 5-7 iulie ,Constanta, Romania, ExPonto Press, 2012, ed. V.Ciupina Si I.M.Stanescu, ISBN978-606-598-181-2, p.149.

[22]Maria Zoran, **Mariana Rodica Didă**, AlexandraTeodora Zoran , Liviu Florin Zoran, Adrian Didă, Outdoor 222Radon concentrations monitoring in relation with particulate matter levels and possible health effects, ISI Journal of Radioanalytical and Nuclear Chemistry, (2013), 296(3), 1179-1192.

[23]Maria Zoran, **Mariana Rodica Didă**, Roxana Savastru, Dan Savastru, Adrian Dida, Ovidiu Ionescu, Ground level ozone (O$_3$) associated with radon (^{222}Rn) and particulate matter (PM) concentrations in Bucharest metropolitan area and adverse health effects, ISI Journal of Radioanalytical and Nuclear Chemistry, (2014), 300, 729-746.

[24]**Didă MR,** M. A. Zoran Satellite and in-Situ monitoring of urban air pollution in relation with children"s asthma", ISI Proc SPIE Proceedings Vol. 8893 ,Earth Resources and Environmental Remote Sensing/GIS Applications IV, Ulrich Michel; Daniel L. Civco; Karsten Schulz,DOI: 10.1117/12.2028737, (2013), November.

[25] **Didă Mariana Rodica**, Maria Zoran, Climate change and extreme heat events in urban areas in relation with Health", Book of Abstracts -13th International Balkan Workshop on Applied Physics Constanța, Romania, July 4-6, (2013), 157.

[26]Zoran M Maria, **Mariana Rodica Didă**, Assessment of the aerosols distribution in the Bucharest metropolitan area inh relation with health effects, ISI SPIE Proc.Micro- to Nano-

Photonics III, ROMOPTO 2012, 10th International Conference on Optics, 3-6 Sept. 2012, Bucuresti, Romania, Conference Proceedings, (2012), 39.

[27]Malik Hamood Ur-Rehman, Kumar K, Frieri Marianne. Minimal Difference in the Prevalence of Asthma in the Urban and Rural Environment Clinical Medicine Insights: Pediatrics ,(2012),6 ,33–39.

[28] Peter Franklin, Merci Kusel. Environmental Contributions to Childhood Asthma Journal of Environmental Immunology and Toxicology, May/June (2013), 1:2, 53-57.

[29]Anne E. Dixon, Fernando Holguin, Akshay Sood, Cheryl M. Salome, Richard E. Pratley, David A. Beuther,Juan C. Celedo´ n, Stephanie A. Shore . An Official American Thoracic Society Workshop Report: Obesity and Asthma, on behalf of the American Thoracic Society Ad Hoc Subcommittee on Obesity and Lung Disease Proc Am Thorac Soc., (2010), 7, 325–335.

[30]Taylor B, Mannino D, Brown C, Crocker D, Twum-Baah N, Holguin F. Body mass index and asthma severity in the national asthma survey. Thorax,(2008),63,14–20.

[31] Murphy K. Susan, Hollingsworth JW. "Stress: A PosSible Link between Genetics, Epigenetics, and Childhood Asthma", American Journal of Respiratory and Critical Care Medicine, (2013), 187(6), 563-564.

www.ingramcontent.com/pod-product-compliance
Lightning Source LLC
Chambersburg PA
CBHW081317180526
45170CB00007B/2741